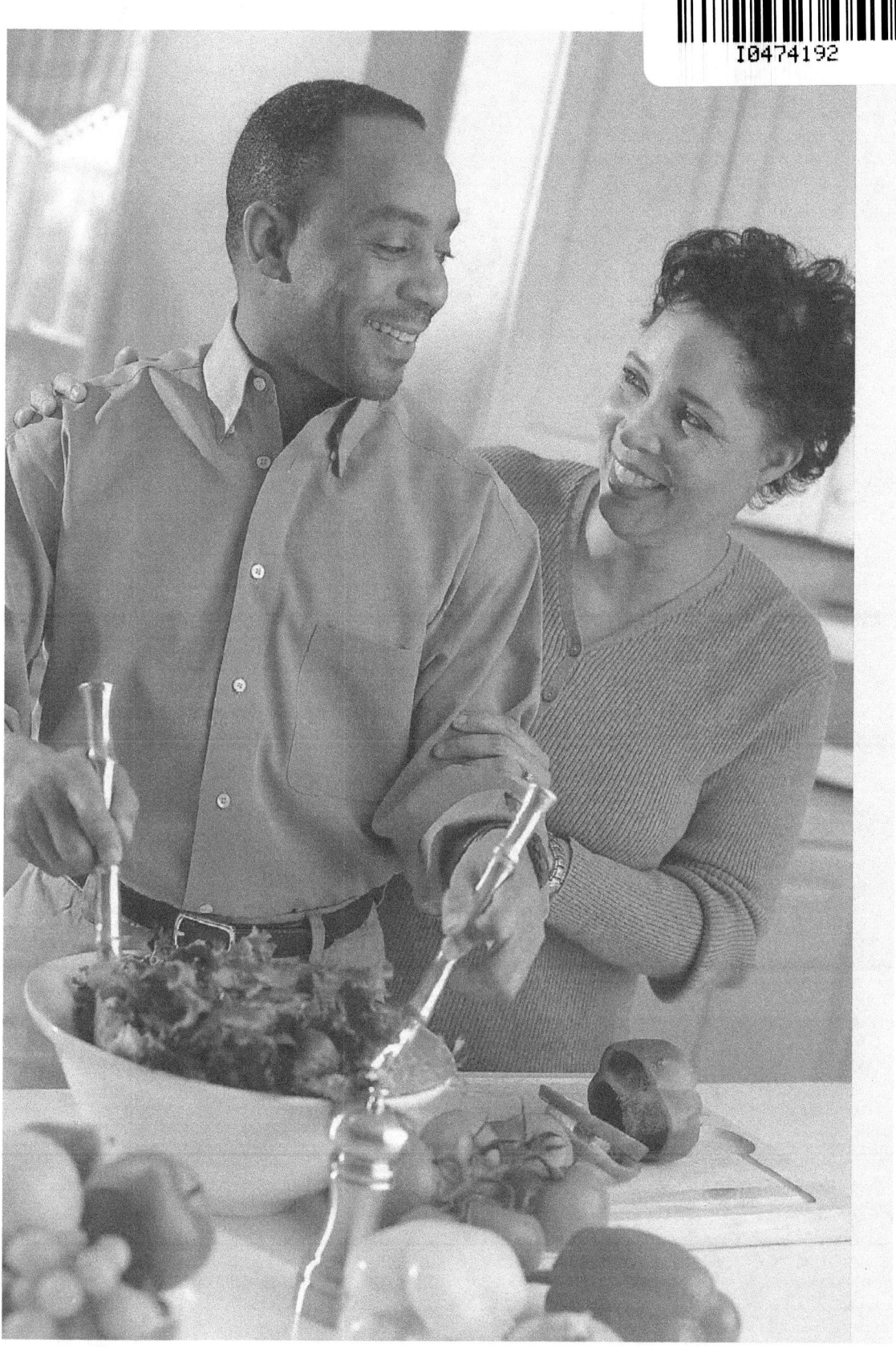

PREFACE

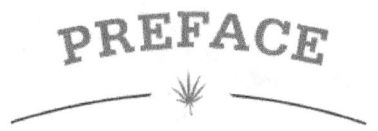

African Americans suffer from higher rates of serious diseases like high blood pressure, Type 2 diabetes, heart disease and some types of cancer. African Americans suffer more serious health problems and die at an earlier age from these diseases. The good news is that eating a healthy diet and leading an active lifestyle promote good health and lowers the chances for getting these illnesses.

A healthy diet includes fruits and vegetables, whole grains, fat-free or low-fat milk products, lean meats, fish, beans, eggs, and nuts. A healthy diet is also low in saturated fat, trans fat, cholesterol, salt and added sugars.

Everyone has the power to make choices to improve his/her health. And eating right doesn't mean giving up our wonderful soul food. In fact, the basic staples of traditional soul food include lots of healthy vegetables: dark leafy greens, sweet potatoes, and high-fiber black eyed peas just to name a few. But they are often cooked with ingredients that add too much saturated fat, calories and salt to our diet.

By making a few simple changes, you and your loved ones can enjoy the flavors of healthy down home cooking. The recipes and hints in this cookbook will help you get started.

TABLE OF CONTENTS

RIGHT STARTS

THE KEY TO COOKING "DOWN HOME HEALTHY" IS A PANTRY STOCKED WITH HEALTHY INGREDIENTS.

INSTEAD OF THIS:	USE THIS:
Ham hocks and fat back	Turkey thighs
Pork bacon	Turkey bacon, lean ham, Canadian bacon
Lard, butter, or other hard fats	Small amount of vegetable oil
Pork sausage	Ground turkey breast
Ground beef and pork	Smoked turkey neck
Neck bone	Skinless chicken thighs
Regular bouillons and broths	Low sodium bouillon and broths
Cream	Evaporated skim milk
Regular cheese	Low fat or lite cheese
High fat cut of beef*	Top round, eye of round, round steak, rump roast, sirloin tip, chuck arm, pot roast, short loin, extra lean ground beef
High fat cut of pork*	Tenderloin, sirloin roast or chop, center cut loin chops
High fat cut of lamb*	Foreshank, leg roast, leg chop, loin chop

* Sometimes less tender cuts of meat like round or rump need marinating. To add flavor and tenderize, use an oil-free marinade. Place meat and marinade in a plastic bag and marinate for 1 to 2 hours in the refrigerator. Throw away the marinade. Don't use it for basing while cooking the meat.

NOW THAT THE PANTRY IS STOCKED,
HERE ARE SOME HEALTHY COOKING TECHNIQUES:

- Steam your vegetables whenever you can. Use garlic, onions, and herbs for flavor. Use very small amounts of butter, cheese, and sauces.

- Use more herbs and spices to flavor greens and other dishes. Cut down on the salt. Try adding Spanish onion and black pepper to black-eyed peas.

- Always use low-fat (1% or 2%) or skim milk for cooking instead of whole milk or cream.

- Put away that deep fat fryer. Try boiling, roasting, baking, grilling, braising, or stir-frying with a little oil instead.

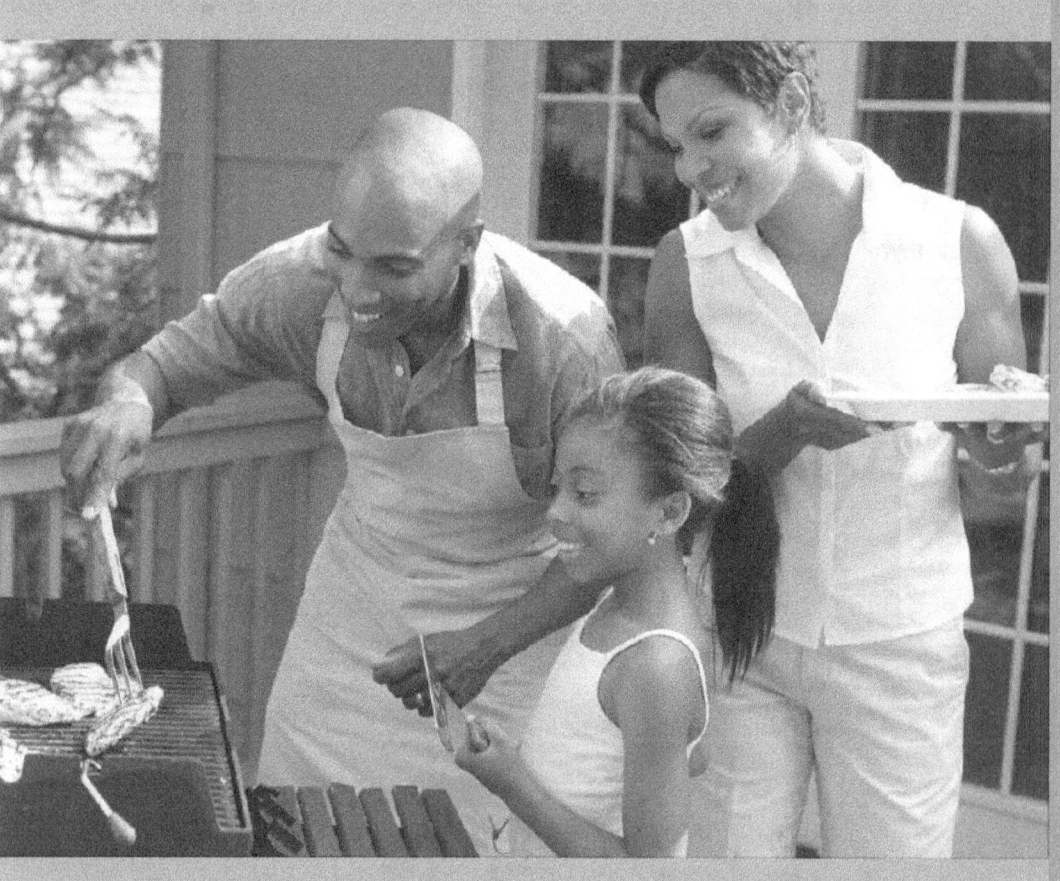

ENTRÉES

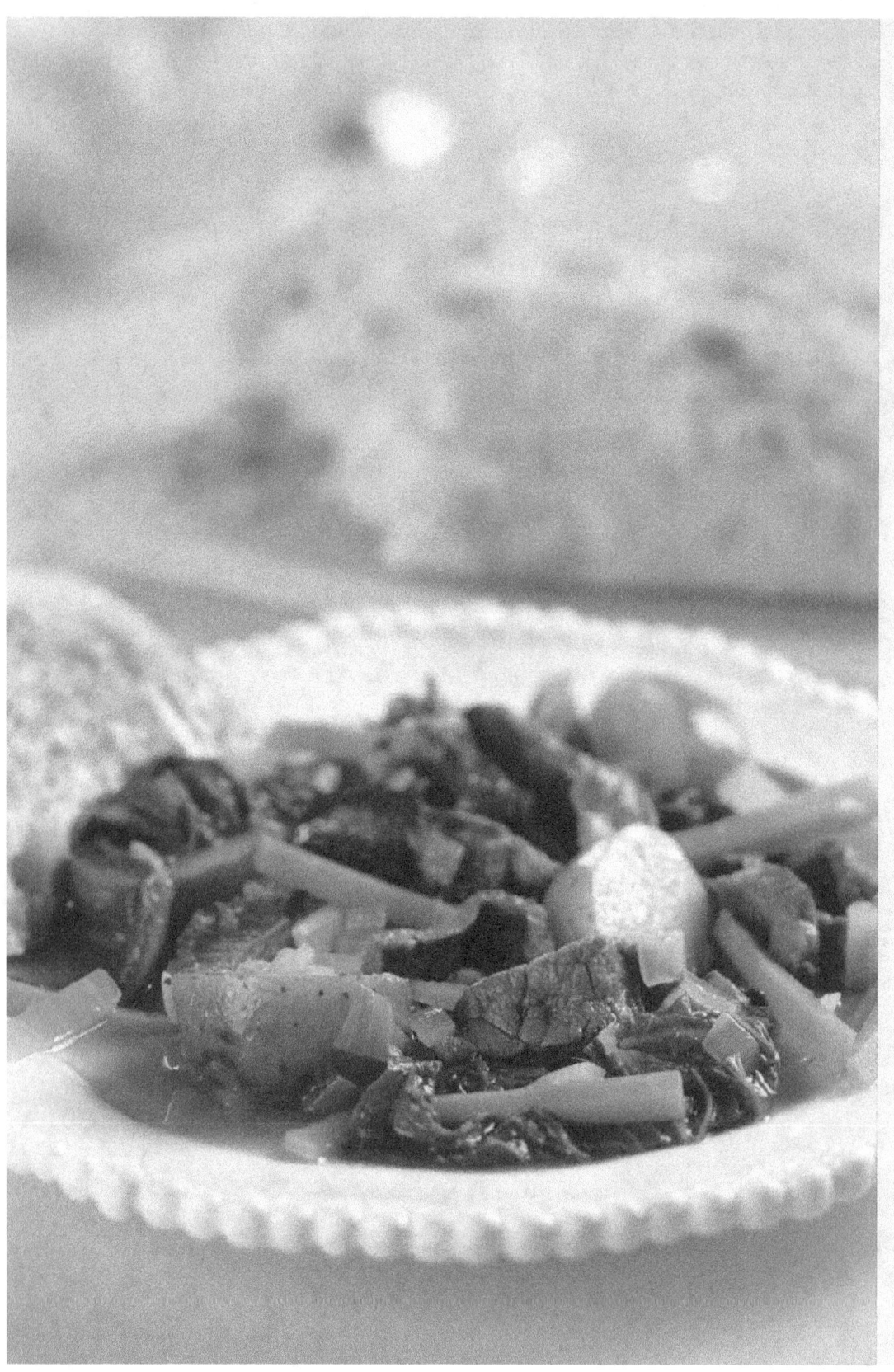

BLACK SKILLET BEEF
with GREENS *and* RED POTATOES

1   Partially freeze beef. Thinly slice across the grain into long strips, 1/8-inch thick. Thoroughly coat strips with Hot 'n Spicy Seasoning.

2   Spray a large, heavy skillet (cast iron is good) with non-stick spray coating. Preheat pan over high heat. Add meat; cook, stirring for 5 minutes.

3   Add potatoes, onion, broth, and garlic. Cook, covered, over medium heat for 20 minutes. Stir in carrots; lay greens over top and cook, covered, until carrots are tender (about 15 minutes). Serve in large serving bowl, with crusty bread for dunking.

INGREDIENTS

1 lb beef top round

1½ tablespoon
Hot 'n Spicy Seasoning
(see recipe on page 19)

8 red-skinned potatoes,
halved

3 cups finely chopped
onion

2 cups beef broth

2 large cloves garlic,
minced

2 large carrots, peeled,
cut into very thin
2½-inch strips

2 bunches (½ lb each)
mustard greens, kale,
or turnip greens, stems
removed, coarsely torn

non-stick cooking spray

CATFISH STEW
with RICE

INGREDIENTS

2 medium potatoes

1, 14½-ounce can
tomatoes, cut up

1 cup chopped onion

1, 8-ounce bottle (1
cup) clam juice or water

1 cup water

2 cloves garlic, minced

½ head cabbage,
coarsely chopped

1 lb catfish fillets

1½ tablespoon
Hot 'n Spicy Seasoning
(see recipe on page 19)

sliced green onion for
garnish (optional)

2 cups hot, cooked rice
(white or brown)

1   Peel potatoes and cut into quarters. In a large pot, combine potatoes, tomatoes and their juice, onion, clam juice, water, and garlic. Bring to boiling; reduce heat. Cook, covered, over medium-low heat for 10 minutes.

2   Add cabbage. Return to boiling. Reduce heat; cook, covered, over medium-low heat for 5 minutes, stirring occasionally.

3   Meanwhile, cut fillets into 2-inch lengths. Coat with Hot 'n Spicy Seasoning. Add fish to vegetables. Reduce heat; simmer, covered, for 5 minutes or until fish flakes easily with a fork.

4   Serve in soup plates, garnished with sliced green onion. Top with an ice cream scoop of hot, cooked rice. Or, ladle stew over hot, cooked rice in soup plates and garnish with green onion.

 To reduce sodium, try low-sodium
canned tomatoes.

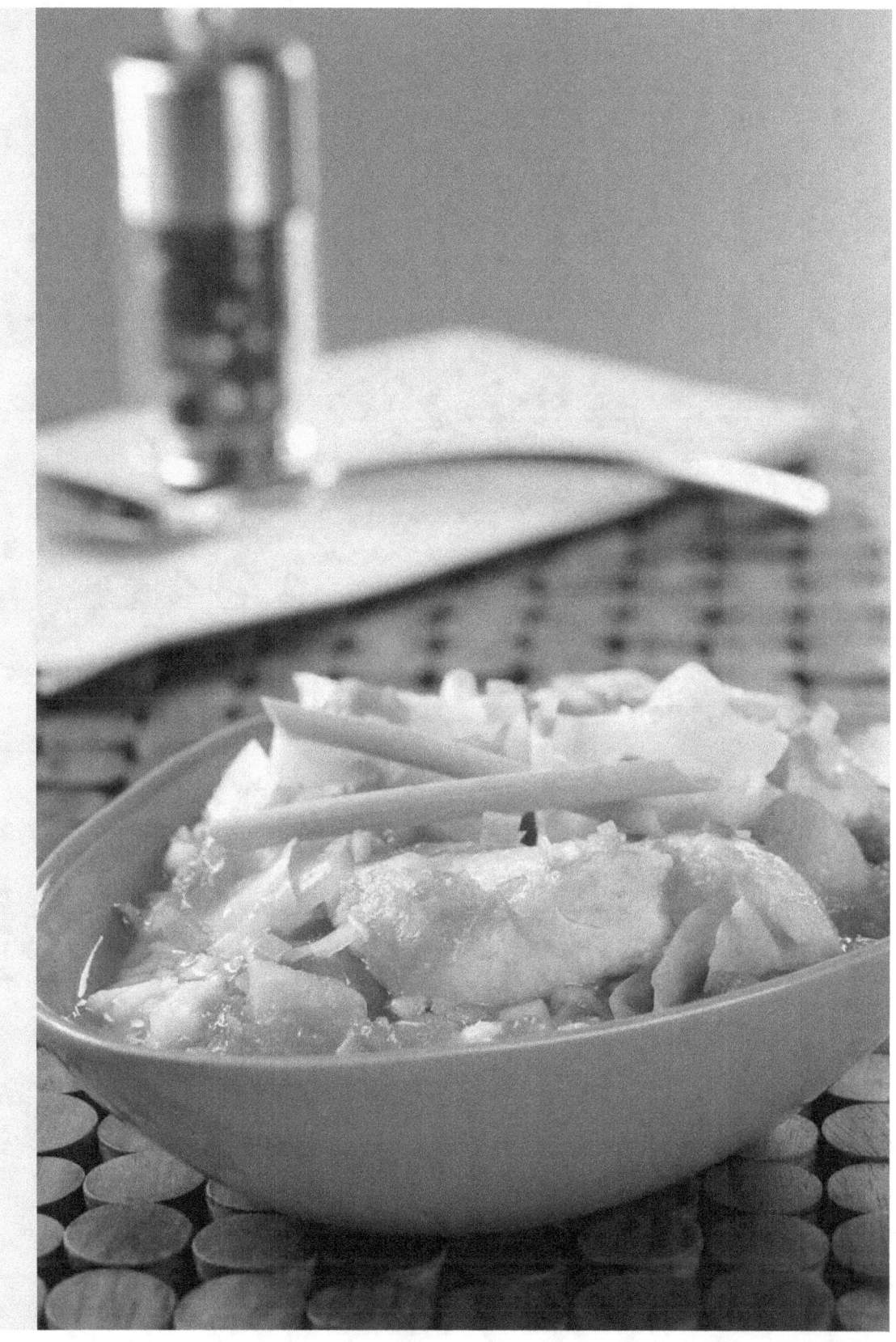

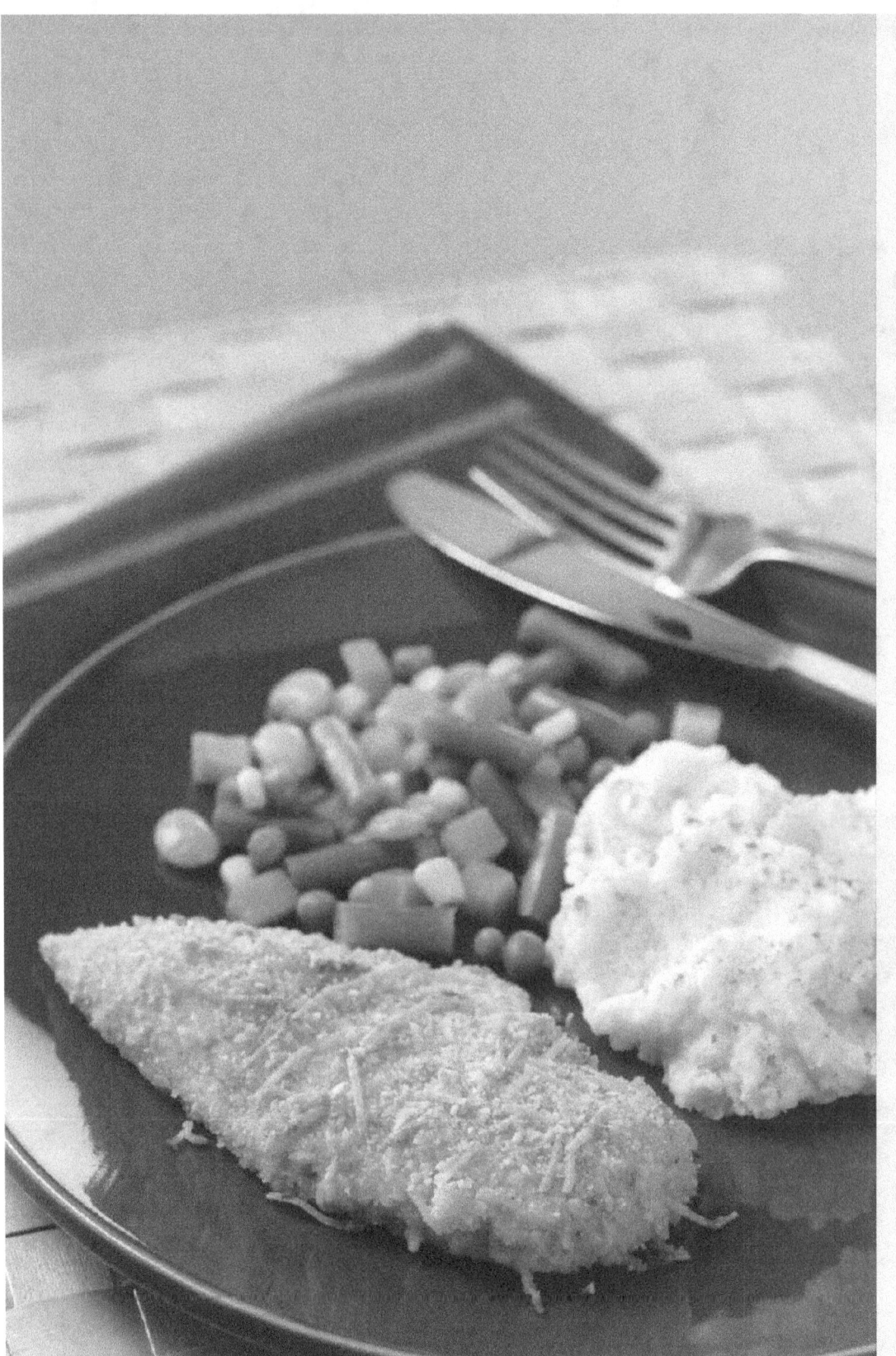

NUTRITION CONTENT
Per Serving
Makes 6 servings

calories: 245
total fat: 5.69g
saturated fat: 2.33g
carbohydrates: 21.09g
protein: 25.8g
cholesterol: 56.61mg
sodium: 476mg
dietary fiber: 4.56g

BAKED FRIED CHICKEN BREAST
with MIXED VEGETABLES

1   Pre-heat oven to 350°. Spray a medium baking pan with cooking spray. On waxed paper, mix bread crumbs, cheese, cornmeal, and ground red pepper.

2   In pie plate, beat egg white and salt. Dip each piece of chicken in egg white mixture, then coat with bread crumb mixture. Place chicken in pan; spray lightly with cooking spray.

3   Bake chicken for 30 minutes or until coating is crisp and juices run clear when chicken is pierced with the tip of a knife. Add mixed vegetables to chicken. Bake for 5 more minutes. Serve with garlic mashed potatoes (page 28).

INGREDIENTS

non-stick cooking spray

½ cup plain dried bread crumbs

½ cup grated Parmesan cheese

2 tablespoons cornmeal

½ teaspoon ground red pepper

1 large egg white

½ teaspoon salt

1½ lbs boneless, skinless chicken breast

3 cups mixed vegetables

NUTRITION CONTENT
Per Serving
Makes 4 servings

calories: 255
total fat: 3g
saturated fat: 0.8g
carbohydrates: 16g
protein: 31g
cholesterol: 100mg
sodium: 465mg
dietary fiber: 1.5g

20-MINUTE
CHICKEN CREOLE

INGREDIENTS

4 medium chicken breast halves
(1½ lbs total) skinned, boned, and cut into 1-inch strips

1, 14-ounce can tomatoes, cut up

1 cup low-sodium chili sauce

1½ cups chopped green pepper (1 large)

½ cup chopped celery

¼ cup chopped onion

2 cloves garlic, minced

1 tablespoon chopped fresh basil or 1 teaspoon dried basil, crushed

1 tablespoon chopped fresh parsley or 1 teaspoon dried parsley

¼ teaspoon crushed red pepper

¼ teaspoon salt

non-stick cooking spray

1   Spray deep skillet with non-stick spray coating. Preheat pan over high heat. Cook chicken in hot skillet, stirring for 3 to 5 minutes or until no longer pink.

2   Reduce heat. Add tomatoes and their juice, low-sodium chili sauce, green pepper, celery, onion, garlic, basil, parsley, crushed red pepper, and salt. Bring to boiling; reduce heat and simmer covered for 10 minutes. Serve over hot, cooked rice or whole wheat pasta.

 To reduce sodium, try low-sodium canned tomatoes.

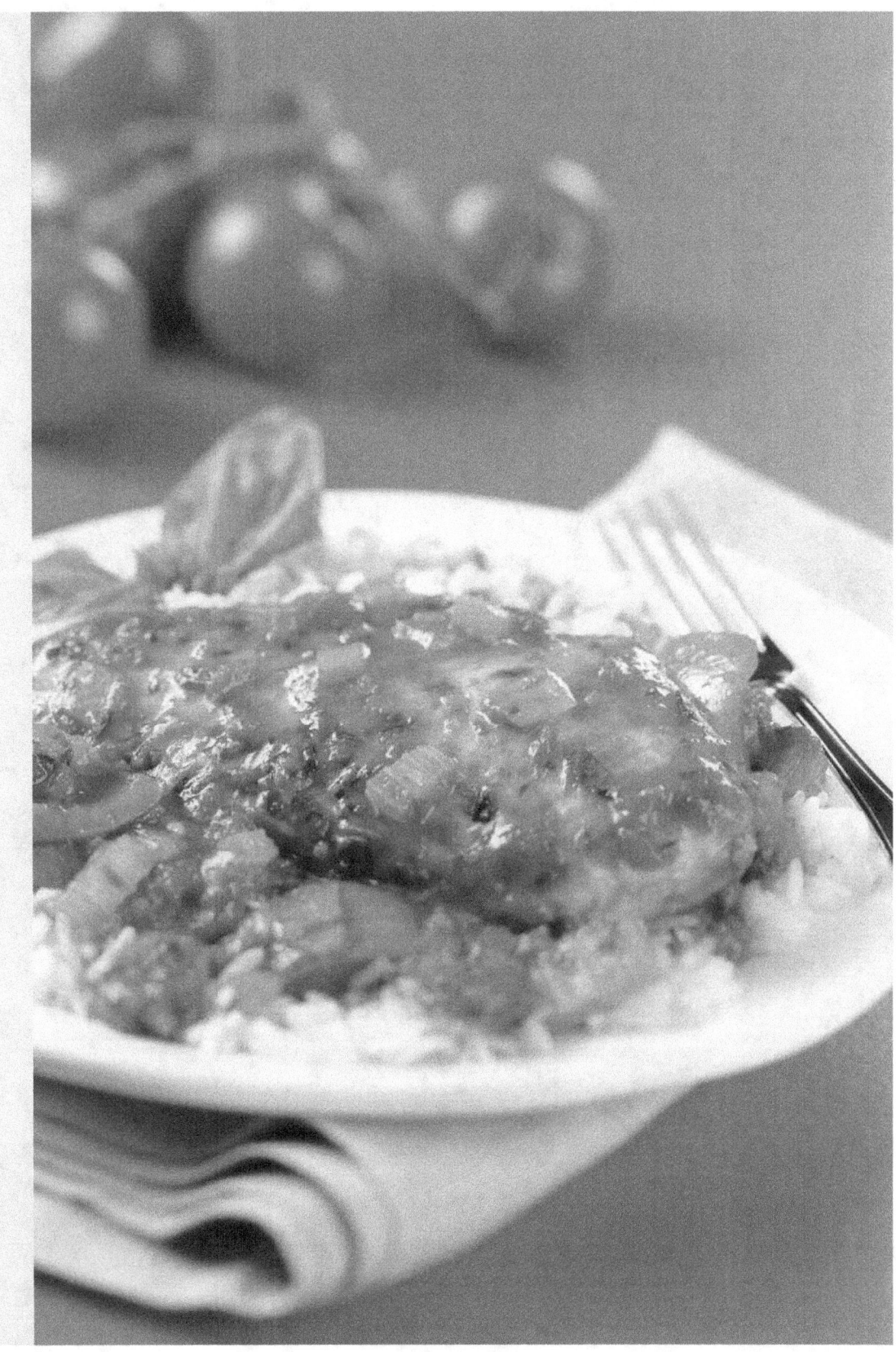

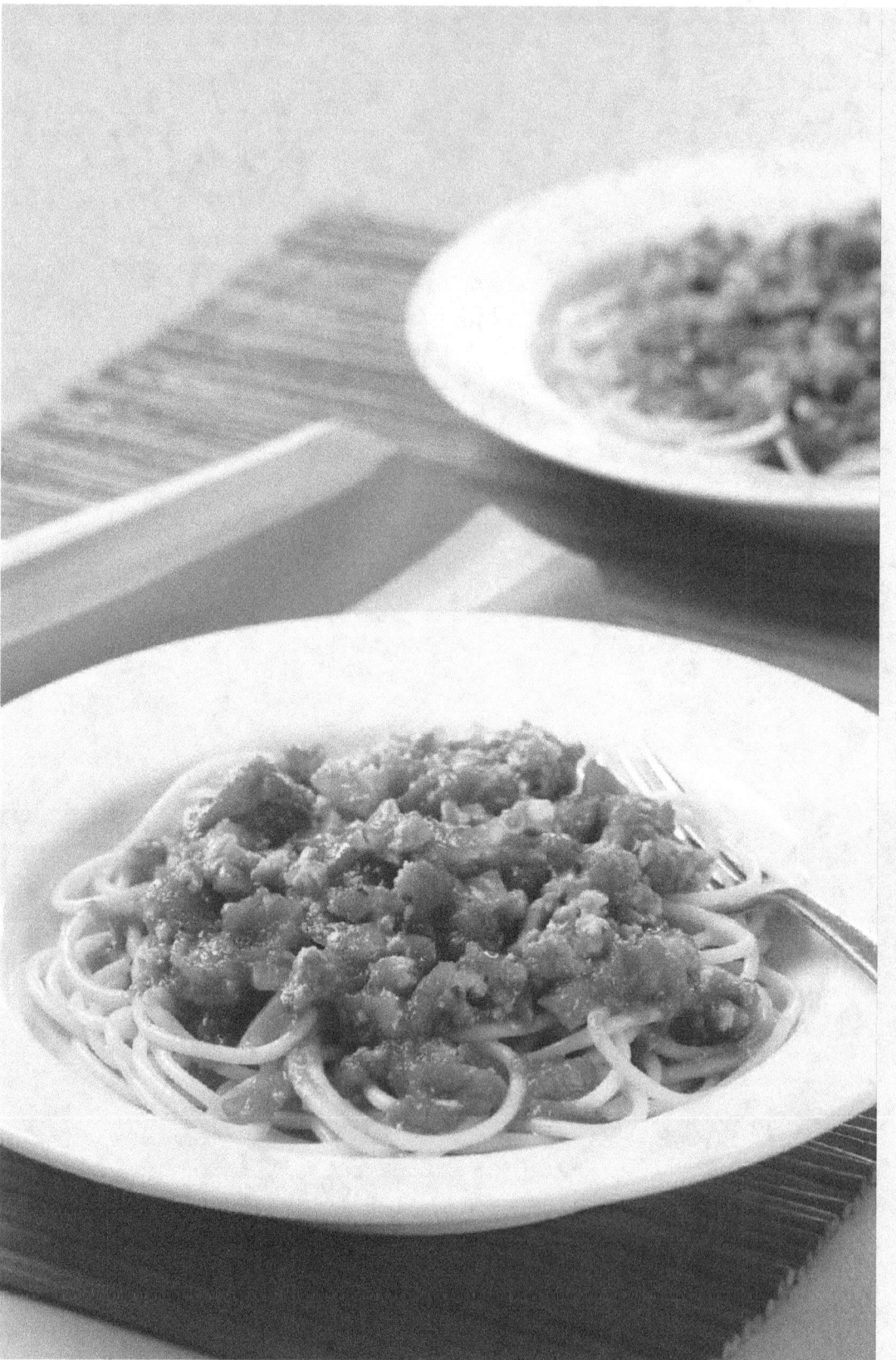

SPAGHETTI
with TURKEY MEAT SAUCE

1. Spray a large skillet with non-stick spray coating. Preheat over high heat. Add turkey; cook, stirring occasionally, for 5 minutes. Drain fat.

2. Stir in tomatoes with their juice, green pepper, onion, garlic, oregano, and black pepper. Bring to boiling; reduce heat. Simmer, covered, for 15 minutes, stirring occasionally.

3. Remove cover; simmer for 15 minutes more. (For a creamier sauce, give sauce a whirl in a blender or food processor.)

4. Meanwhile, cook spaghetti according to package directions; drain well. Serve sauce over spaghetti with crusty, whole-grain bread.

INGREDIENTS

1 lb ground turkey

1, 28-ounce can tomatoes, cut up

1 cup finely chopped green pepper

1 cup finely chopped onion

2 cloves garlic, minced

1 teaspoon dried oregano, crushed

1 teaspoon black pepper

1 lb spaghetti

non-stick cooking spray

NUTRITION CONTENT
Per Serving
Makes 6 servings

calories: 186
total fat: 4.9g
saturated fat: 1.8g
carbohydrates: 16g
protein: 17g
cholesterol: 31mg
sodium: 393mg
dietary fiber: 0.2 g

BAKED
PORK CHOPS

INGREDIENTS

6 lean center–cut pork chops, ½ inch thick

1 egg white

1 cup evaporated skim milk

¾ cup cornflake crumbs

1¼ cup fine dry bread crumbs

2 tablespoons Hot 'n Spicy Seasoning (see recipe on page 19)

1½ teaspoon salt

nonstick spray coating

1 Trim all fat from chops.

2 Beat egg white with evaporated skim milk. Place chops in milk mixture; let stand for 5 minutes, turning chops once.

3 Meanwhile, mix together cornflake crumbs, bread crumbs, Hot 'n Spicy Seasoning and salt. Remove chops from milk mixture. Coat thoroughly with crumb mixture.

4 Spray a 13-inch x 9-inch baking pan with nonstick spray coating. Place chops in pan; bake in 375° oven for 20 minutes. Turn chops; bake 15 minutes longer or until no pink remains.

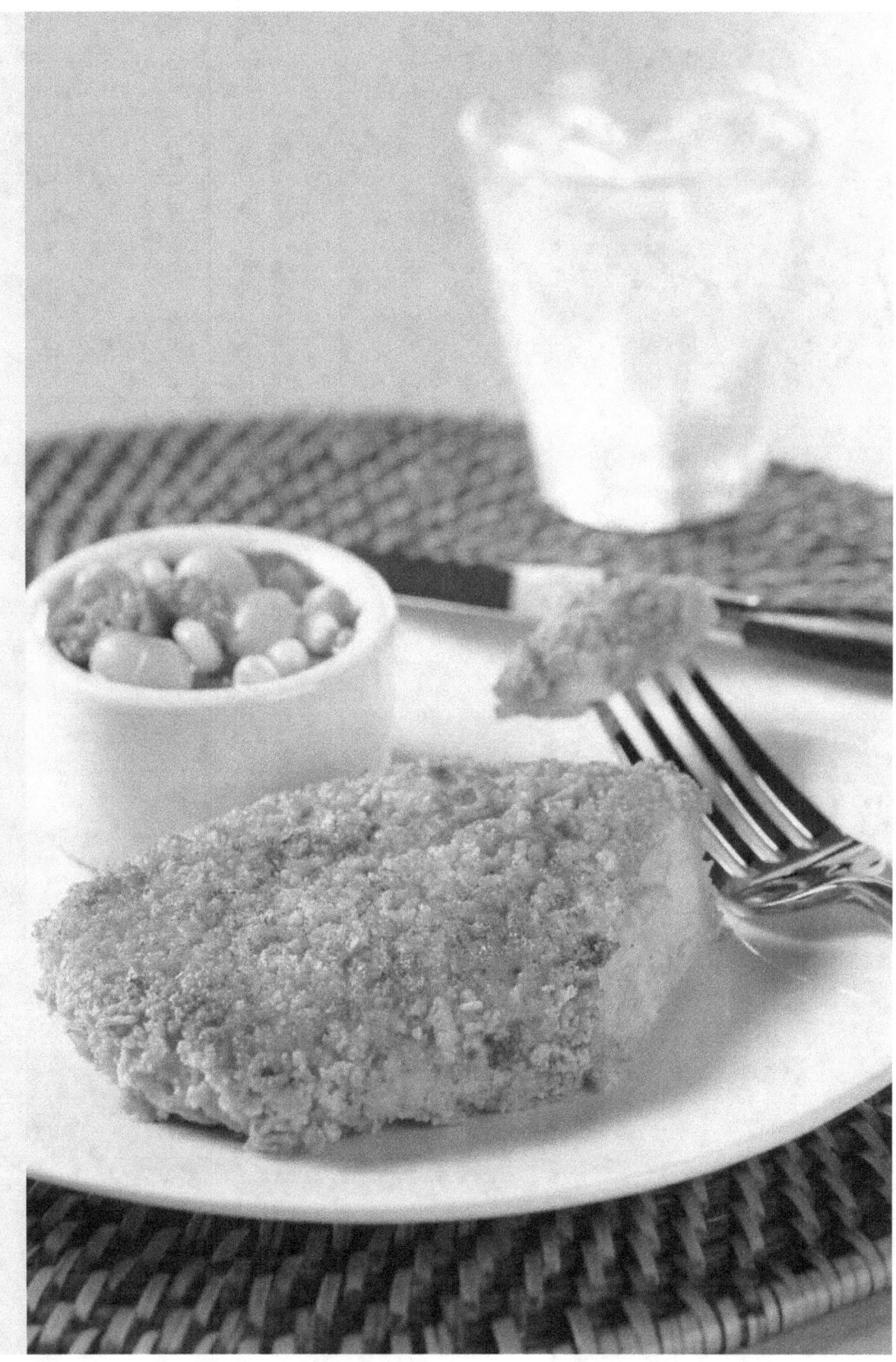

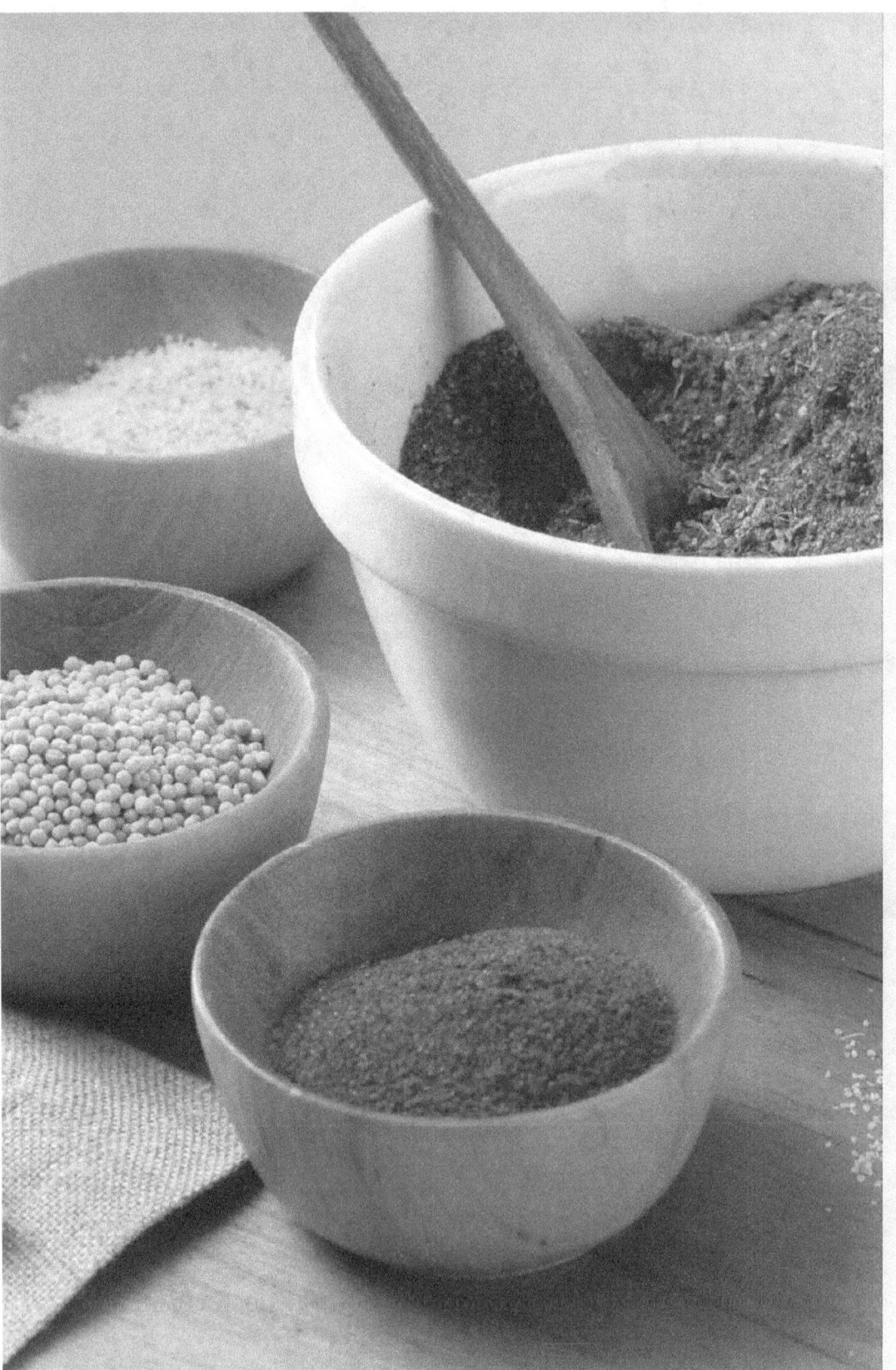

HOT'N SPICY
SEASONING

Mix together all ingredients. Store in airtight container.

Makes about $1/3$ cup.

¼ cup paprika

2 tablespoons
dried oregano, crushed

2 teaspoons
chili powder

1 teaspoon
garlic powder

1 teaspoon
black pepper

½ teaspoon
red (cayenne) pepper

½ teaspoon dry mustard

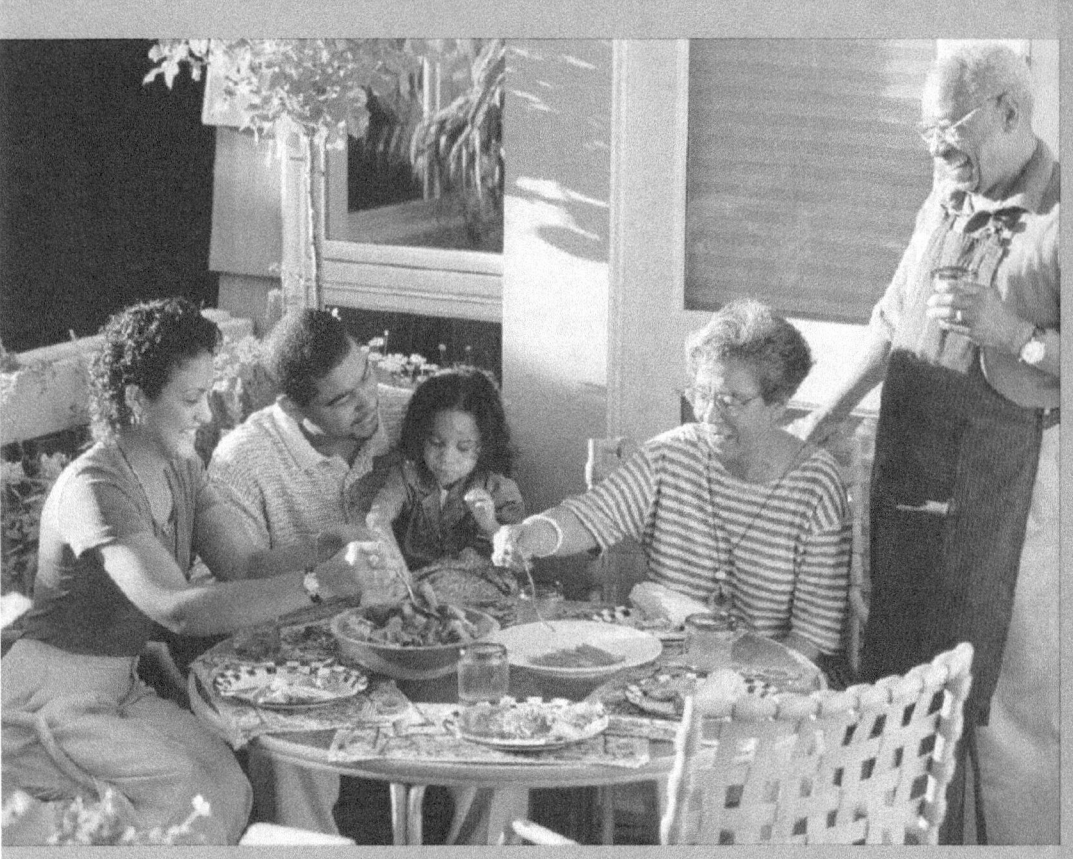

SIDES

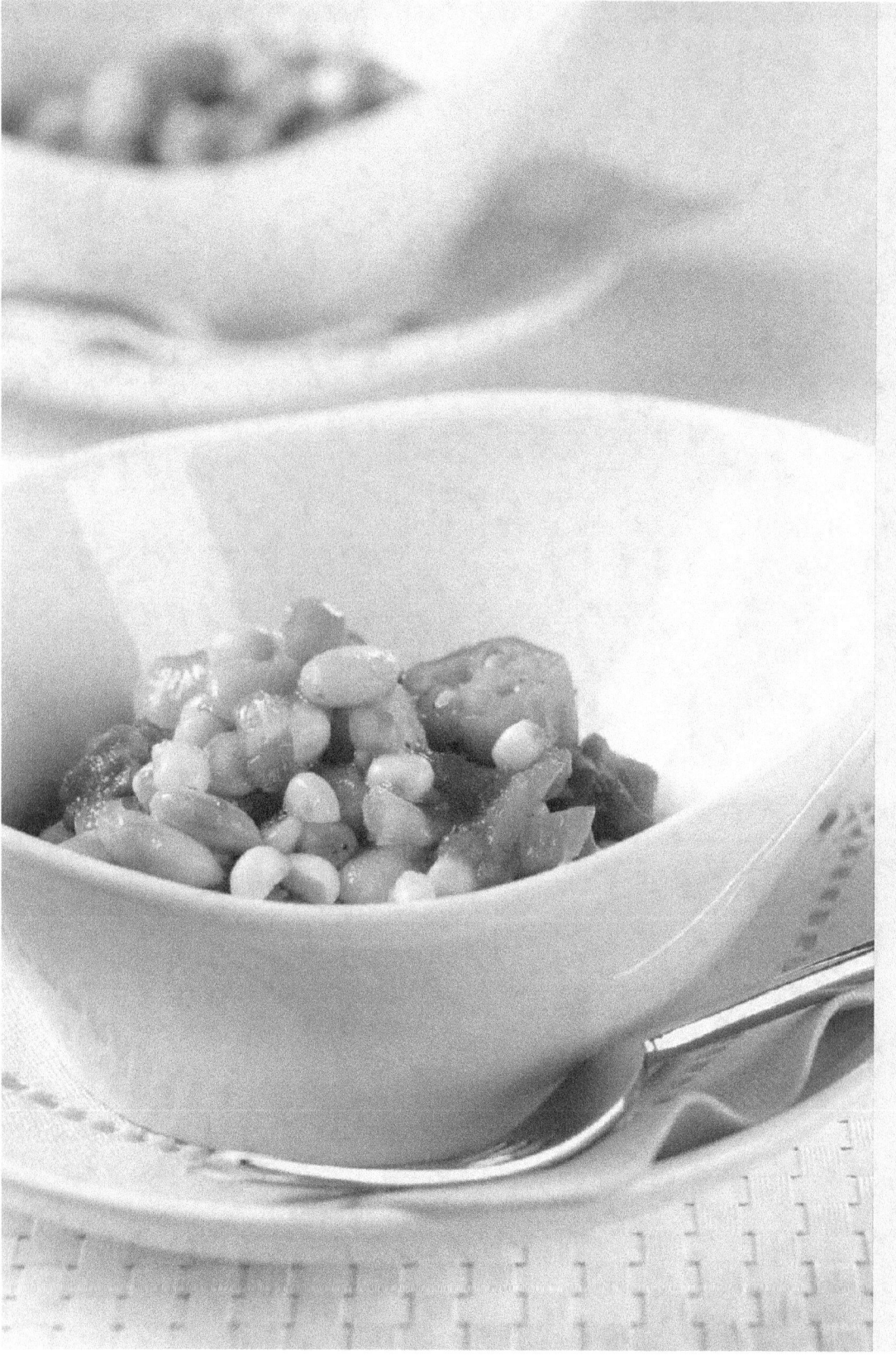

NUTRITION CONTENT
Per Serving
Makes 6 servings

calories: 146
total fat: 3.44g
saturated fat: 0.77g
carbohydrates: 26.05g
protein: 5.89g
cholesterol: 0mg
sodium: 363mg
dietary fiber: 6.16g

SUCCOTASH

1   Combine lima beans, margarine, corn, tomatoes, onions, Tabasco sauce, salt, and pepper in a pan.

2   Bring to a boil, reduce heat, and simmer for 20 minutes.

3   Add okra and cook for 10 more minutes.

INGREDIENTS

10-ounce baby lima beans (frozen)

2 tablespoons margarine (such as Promise™ 60% spread)

10-ounce whole kernel corn (frozen)

10-ounce cut okra

15-ounce canned tomatoes (undrained)

½ cup chopped onions

Tabasco sauce to taste

Salt and black pepper to taste

 This recipe is packed with fiber. Fiber is the part of plant foods that your body can't digest. Beans, most fruits and vegetables, whole grain products, and nuts and seeds are good sources of fiber. Soluble fiber can help lower cholesterol. It also slows down digestion so that the body can absorb more nutrients and better control blood sugar levels. Insoluble fiber helps you get rid of waste and keeps you regular.

NEW ORLEANS
RED BEANS

INGREDIENTS

1 lb dry red beans

2 quarts water

1½ cups chopped onion

1 cup chopped celery

4 bay leaves

1 cup chopped sweet
green pepper

3 tablespoons
chopped garlic

3 tablespoons
chopped parsley

2 teaspoons dried
thyme, crushed

1 teaspoon salt

1 teaspoon
black pepper

1   Pick through beans to remove bad beans; rinse thoroughly. In a 5-quart pot, combine beans, water, onion, celery, and bay leaves. Bring to boiling; reduce heat. Cover and cook over low heat for about 1½ hours or until beans are tender. Stir and mash some of the beans against side of the pan to thicken the mixture.

2   Add green pepper, garlic, parsley, thyme, salt, and black pepper. Cook, uncovered, over low heat until creamy, about 30 minutes. Remove bay leaves.

3   Serve over hot, cooked brown rice, if desired.

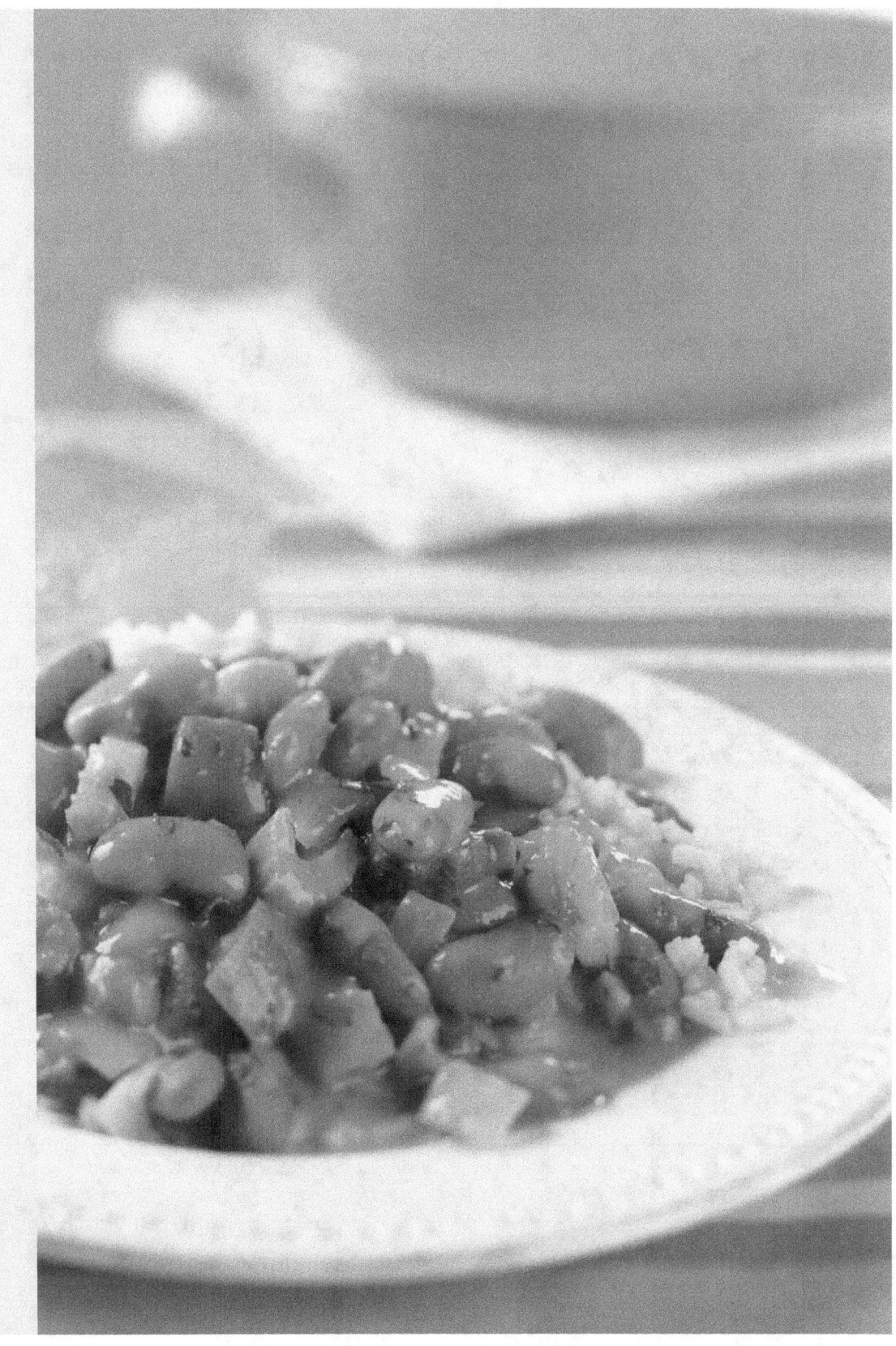

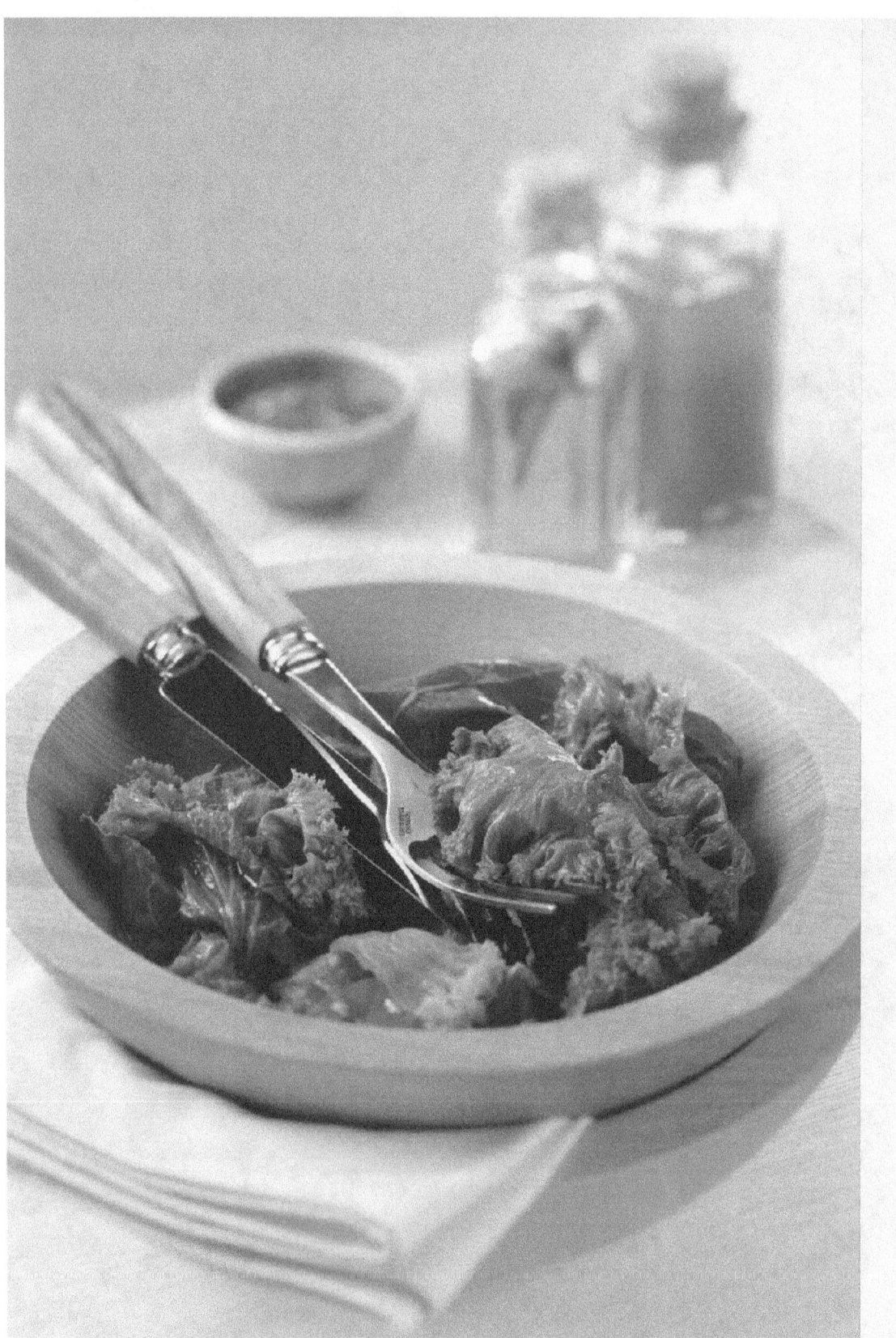

NUTRITION CONTENT
Per Serving
Makes 8 servings

calories: 18
total fat: 0.1g
saturated fat: 0g
carbohydrates: 3g
protein: 1g
cholesterol: 0mg
sodium: 153mg
dietary fiber: 2g

MIXED GREENS

INGREDIENTS

2 bunches mustard greens or kale

2 bunches turnip greens

pepper to taste (optional)

1 teaspoon salt, or to taste (optional)

1   Rinse greens well, removing stems. In a large pot of boiling water, cook greens rapidly, covered, over medium heat for about 25 minutes or until tender.

2   Serve with some of the pot liquor (liquid from the cooked greens). If desired, cut greens in pan with a sharp knife and kitchen fork before serving.

 Beet greens like collards, mustard and turnip greens are a good source of potassium which helps maintain healthy blood pressure. Potassium counteracts the effect of sodium on blood pressure. Too much sodium causes the blood pressure to rise. Dark green leafy vegetables are naturally high in potassium and low in sodium.

GARLIC

MASHED POTATOES

INGREDIENTS

1 lb potatoes (2 large)

2 cups skim milk

2 large cloves garlic, chopped

½ teaspoon white pepper

1   Peel potatoes; cut in quarters. Cook, covered, in a small amount of boiling water for 20 to 25 minutes or until tender. Remove from heat. Drain. Cover the pot.

2   Meanwhile, in a saucepan over low heat, cook garlic in milk until garlic is soft, about 30 minutes.

3   Add milk-garlic mixture and white pepper to potatoes. Beat with an electric mixer on low speed or mash with a potato masher until smooth.

 Use low-fat (1% or 2%) or nonfat/skim milk instead of whole milk.

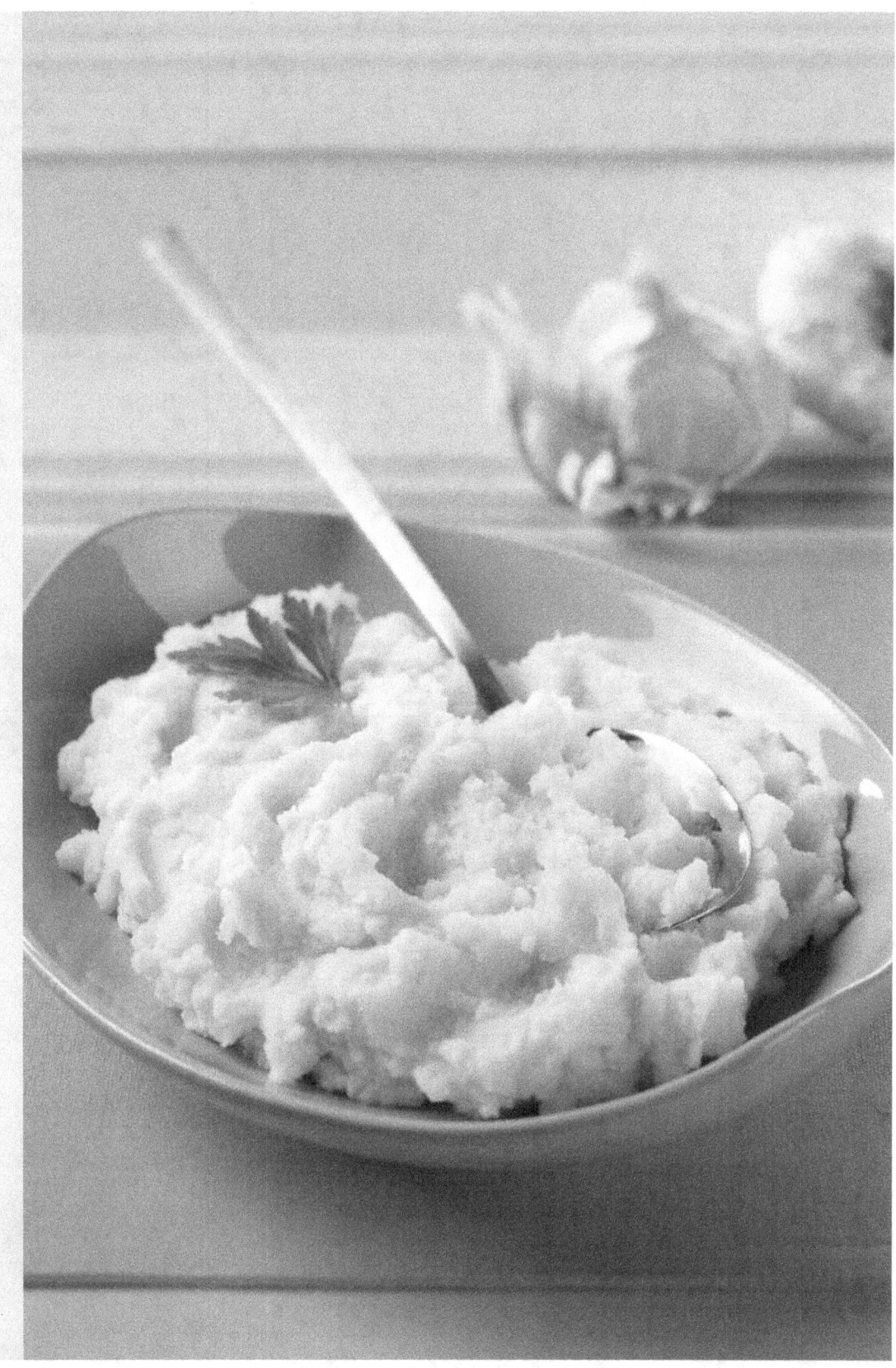

HONEY
CANDIED YAMS

INGREDIENTS

3 small yams

¼ cup honey

½ cup water

¼ teaspoon ground nutmeg

1 tablespoon light margarine

¼ teaspoon lemon flavor

1   Wash and peel yams. Cut in quarters and then cut into 2 pieces each. Rinse pieces.

2   Place yams, honey, water, nutmeg, margarine, and flavor in a sauce pan and heat until boiling.

3   Turn heat down to medium, cover and let simmer until all water boils out and the sauce is syrupy.

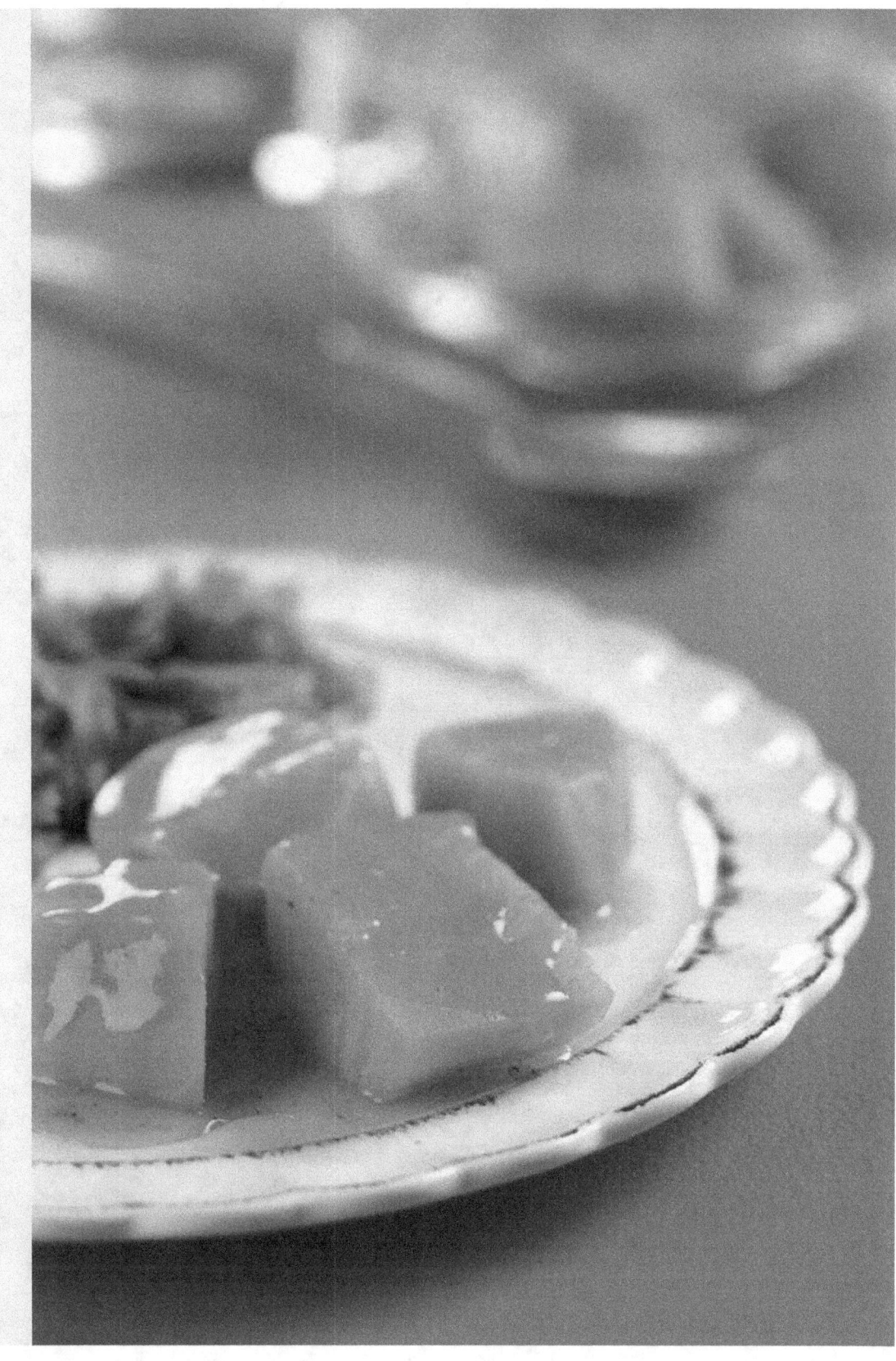

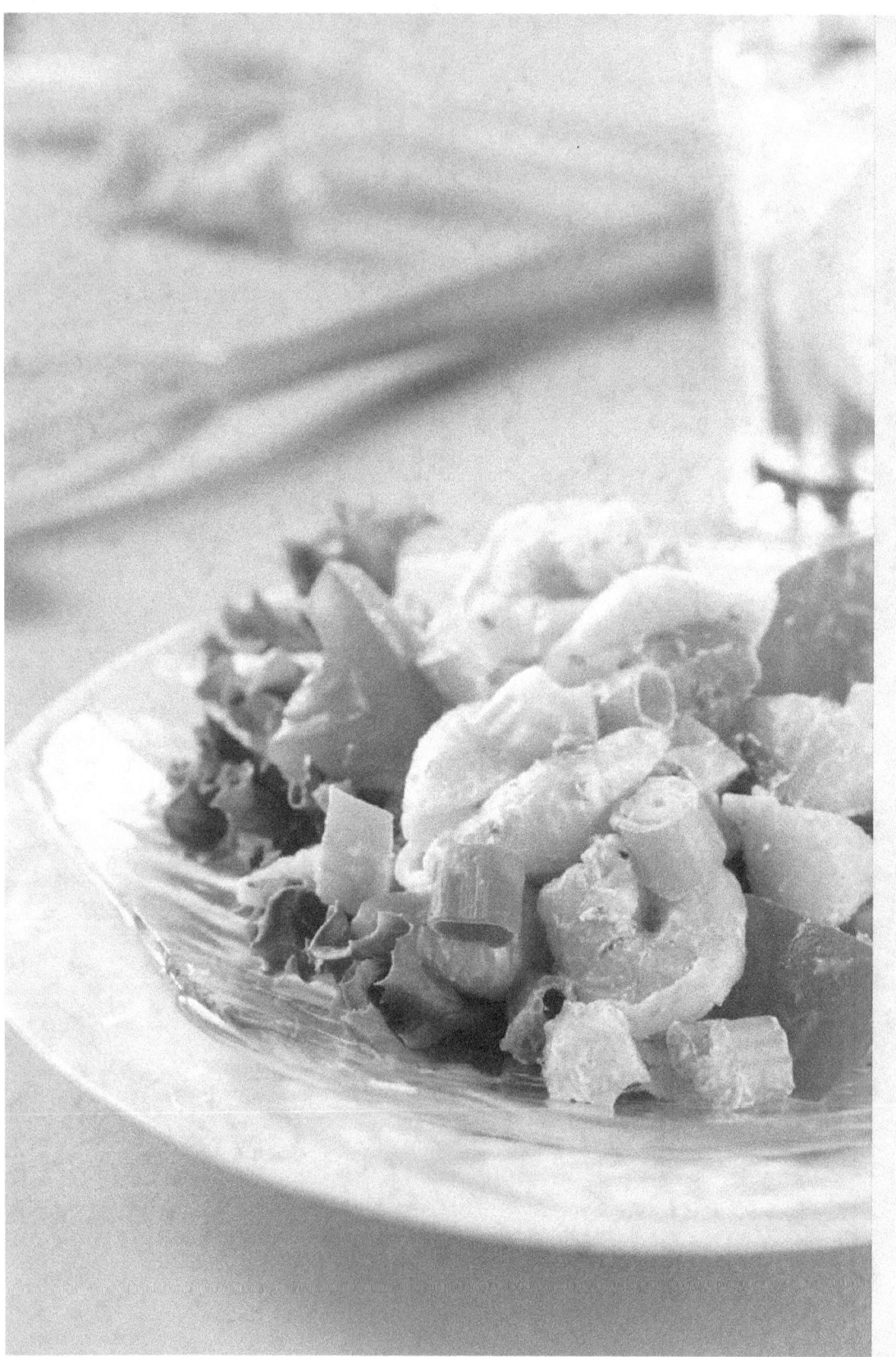

NUTRITION CONTENT
Per Serving
Makes 12 servings

calories: 140
total fat: 1g
carbohydrates: 1g
saturated fat: 0.1g
protein: 14g
cholesterol: 60mg
sodium: 135mg
dietary fiber: 1.3g

CHILLIN' OUT
PASTA SALAD

1 Cook pasta according to package directions. Drain; cool.

2 In a large bowl stir together yogurt, mustard, and herb seasoning. Add pasta, celery, and green onion; mix well. Chill at least 2 hours.

3 Just before serving, carefully stir in shrimp and tomatoes.

INGREDIENTS

8-ounce (2½ cups) medium shell pasta

1, 8-ounce carton (1 cup) plain nonfat yogurt

2 tablespoons spicy brown mustard

2 tablespoons salt-free herb seasoning

1½ cups chopped celery

1 cup sliced green onion

1 lb cooked small shrimp

3 cups coarsely chopped tomatoes (about 3 large)

GARDEN
POTATO SALAD

INGREDIENTS

3 lbs potatoes (6 large)

1 cup chopped celery

½ cup sliced green onion

2 tablespoons chopped parsley

DRESSING

1 cup low-fat cottage cheese

¾ cup skim milk

3 tablespoons lemon juice

2 tablespoons cider vinegar

½ teaspoon celery seed

½ teaspoon dillweed

½ teaspoon dry mustard

½ teaspoon white pepper

1   In a blender, blend cottage cheese, milk, lemon juice, vinegar, celery seed, dillweed, dry mustard, and white pepper until smooth. Chill for 1 hour.

2   Scrub potatoes; boil in jackets until tender. Cool; peel. Cut into ½-inch cubes. Add celery, green onion, and parsley.

3   Pour chilled cottage cheese mixture over vegetables; mix well. Chill at least 30 minutes before serving.

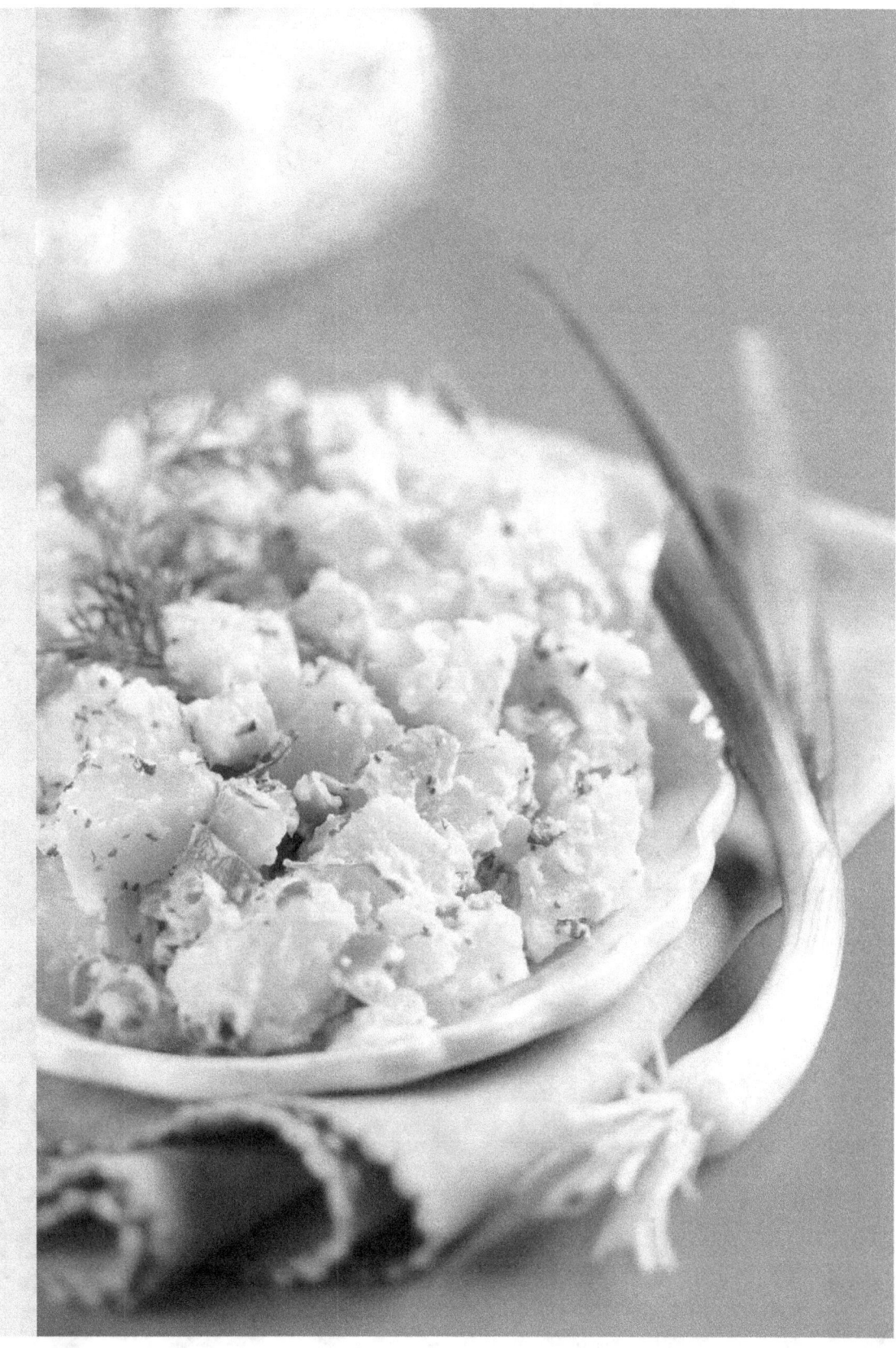

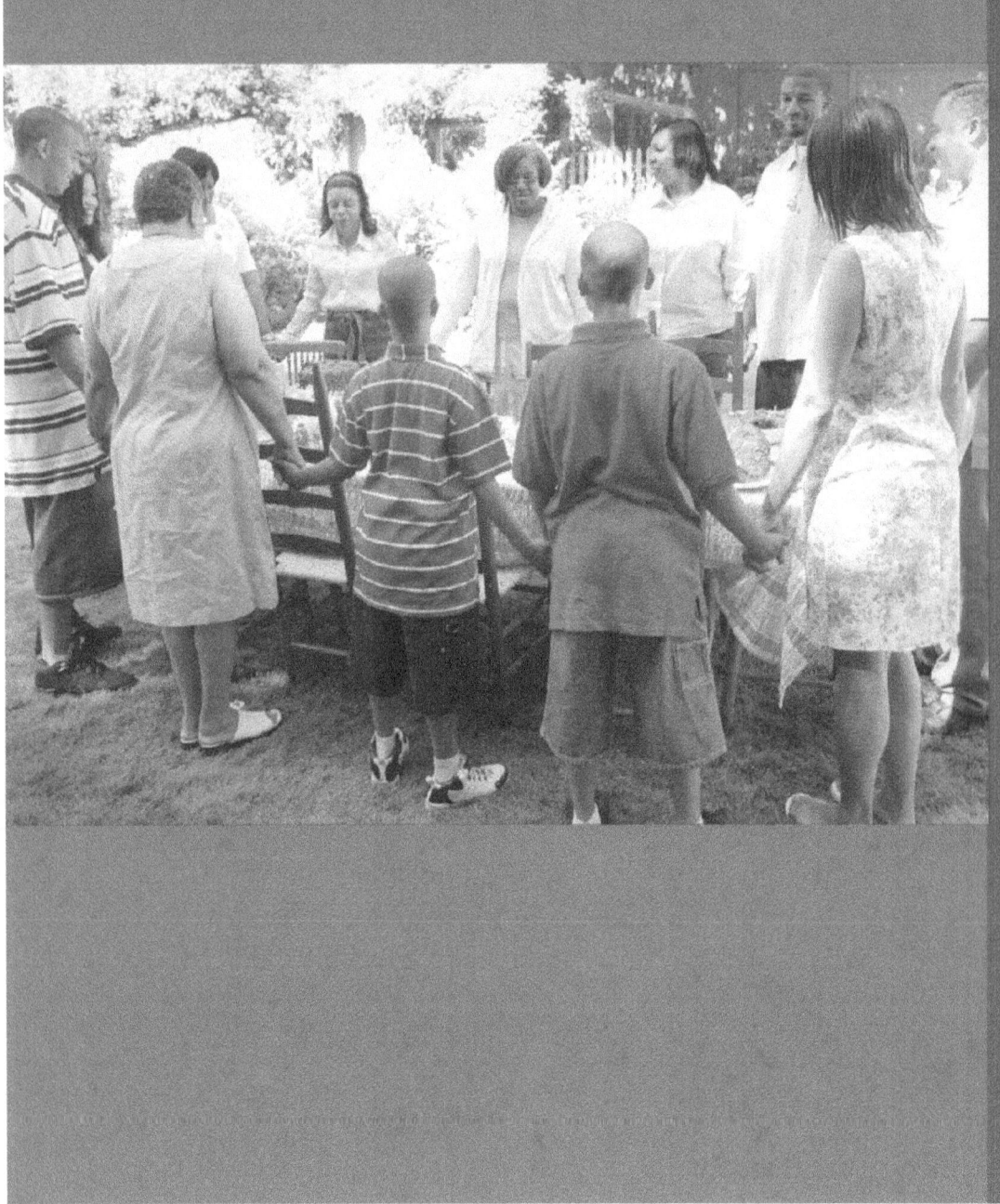

DESSERTS

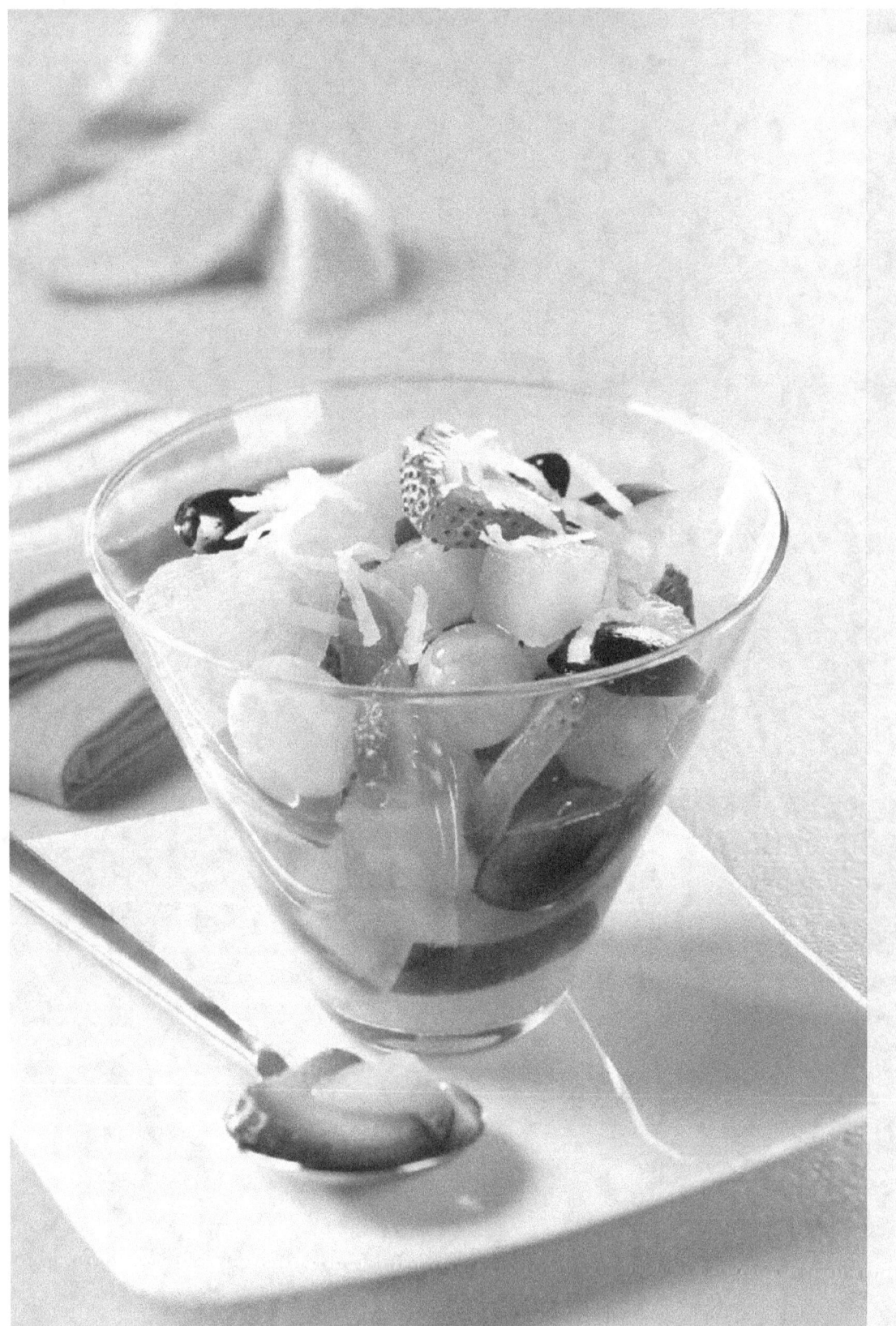

FRUIT SALAD

1   Wash all fresh fruits well. Slice grapes. Slice straw-
    berries and remove stems. Peel orange, slice and
    remove seeds and membranes, and cut into bite-
    size pieces. Peel apples, remove core, and cut into
    small pieces. Combine fruit in large bowl.

2   Add fruit cocktail.

3   Stir until all fruit is mixed. Level the top and sprin-
    kle coconut. Chill. Serve.

INGREDIENTS

1 lb seedless black grapes

6 medium red apples

1 pint strawberries

6 medium oranges

16-ounce can of fruit cocktail, packed in juice

1 cup coconut (shredded)

 Fruits and vegetables provide many important
vitamins, like vitamin A and vitamin C. There are
about 20 vitamins needed for life. The best way to
get them is to eat the fruits and vegetables that
contain them.

WINTER *and* SUMMER CRISP

INGREDIENTS

FILLING

½ cup granulated sugar

3 tablespoons
all-purpose flour

1 teaspoon
grated lemon peel

5 cups unpeeled, sliced
apples

1 cup cranberries

TOPPING

⅔ cup rolled oats

⅓ cup packed brown
sugar

¼ cup whole wheat
flour

2 teaspoons
ground cinnamon

3 tablespoons
soft margarine, melted

1   In a medium bowl, combine sugar, flour, and lemon peel; mix well. Add apples and cranberries; stir to mix. Spoon into a 6-cup baking dish.

2   In a small bowl, combine oats, brown sugar, flour, and cinnamon. Add melted margarine; stir to mix. Sprinkle topping over filling.

3   Bake in a 375° oven for 40 to 50 minutes or until filling is bubbly and top is brown. Serve warm or at room temperature.

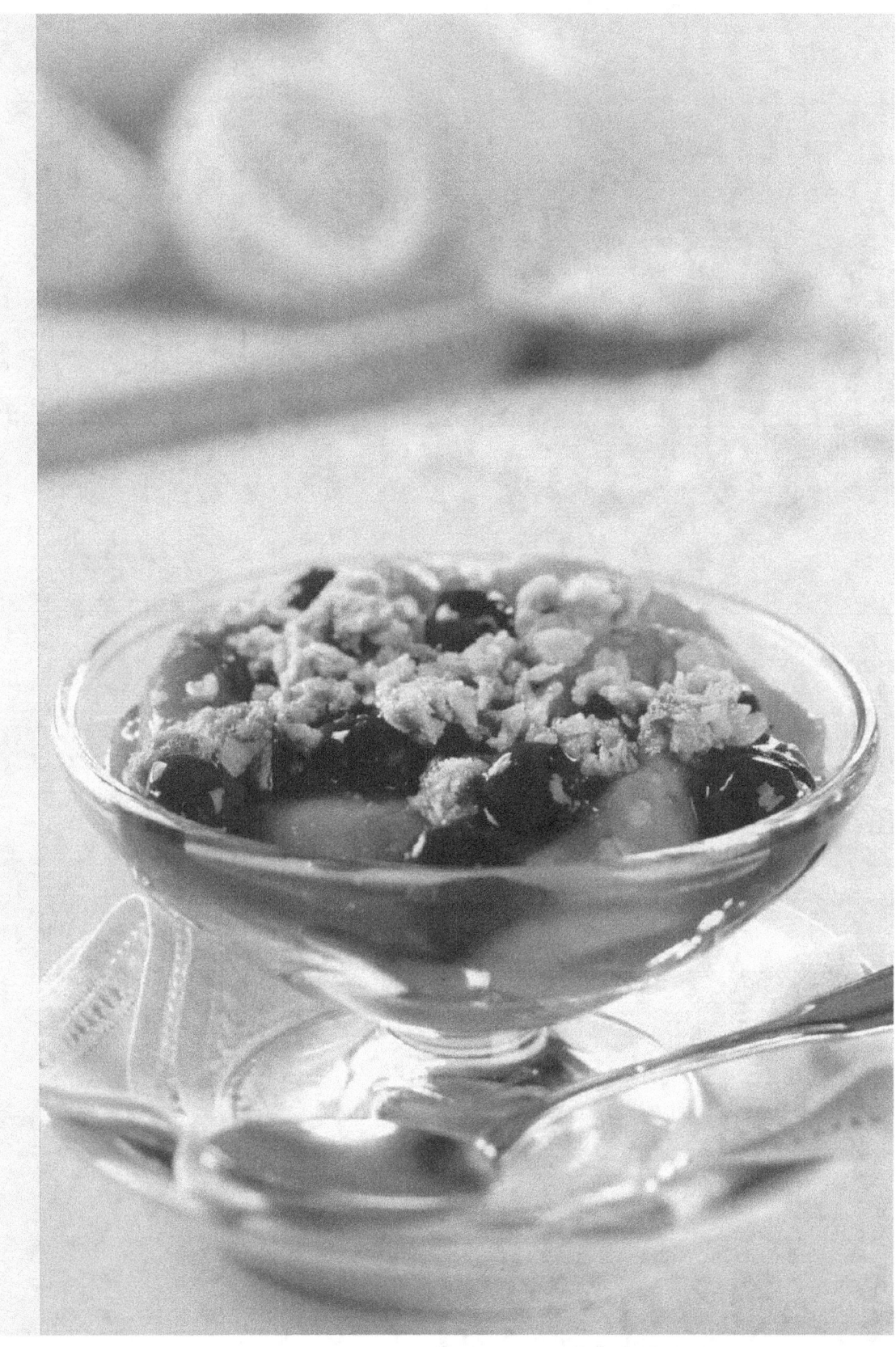

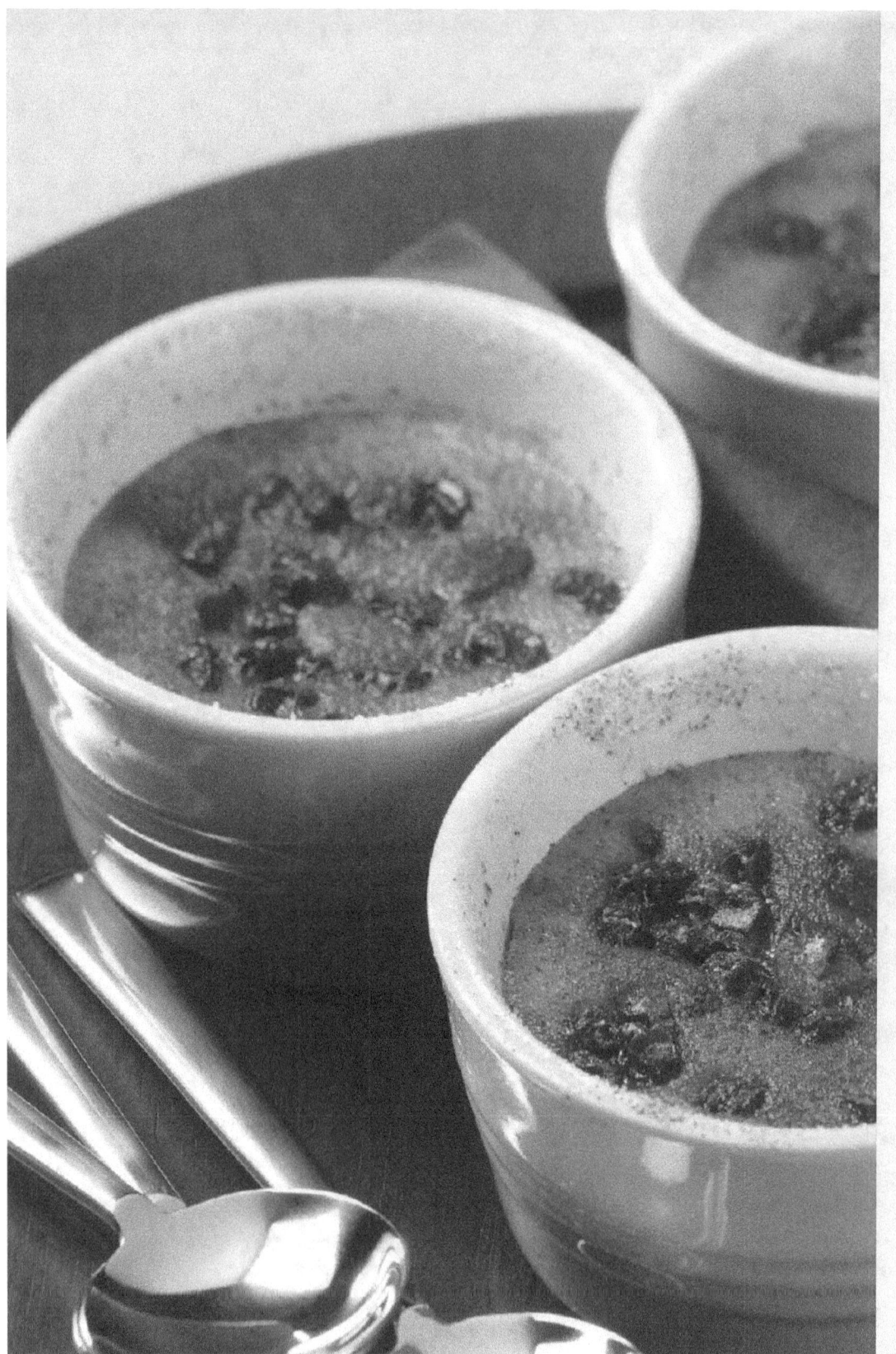

NUTRITION CONTENT
Per Serving
Makes 6 servings

calories: 144
total fat: 2g
saturated fat: 0.7g
carbohydrates: 20g
protein: 6g
cholesterol: 92mg
sodium: 235mg
dietary fiber: 1.4g

SWEET POTATO
CUSTARD

1   In a medium bowl, stir together sweet potato and banana. Add milk, blending well. Add brown sugar, egg yolks, and salt, mixing thoroughly.

2   Spray a 1-quart casserole with non-stick spray coating. Transfer sweet potato mixture to casserole.

3   Combine raisins, sugar, and cinnamon; sprinkle over top of sweet potato mixture. Bake in a preheated 300° F oven for 45 to 50 minutes or until a knife inserted near center comes out clean.

 The deep orange color of sweet potatoes is a sign that they are a good source of vitamin A and the antioxidant beta-carotene. Vitamin A and beta-carotene are good for your skin.

INGREDIENTS

1 cup cooked, mashed sweet potato

½ cup mashed banana (about 2 small)

1 cup evaporated skim milk

2 tablespoons packed brown sugar

2 beaten egg yolks (or 1⅓-cup egg substitute)

½ teaspoon salt

¼ cup raisins

1 tablespoon sugar

1 teaspoon ground cinnamon

Non-stick cooking spray

ANGEL FOOD CAKE
with MIXED BERRIES

INGREDIENTS

1 angel food cake

1 pint blueberries

2 pints strawberries

1 package strawberry glaze (1 cup prepared)

1 pint blackberries

1 lemon (sliced)

1   Bake or buy an angel food cake.

2   Cut tops off one pint of strawberries. Combine with ½ pint of blackberries, ½ pint of blueberries, and strawberry glaze. Reserve remaining berries for garnish.

3   Mix well so that berries are thoroughly coated with glaze.

4   To serve, spoon ½ to ¾ cup of glazed berry mixture over each slice of cake. Garnish each slice with a slice of lemon and a few unglazed berries.

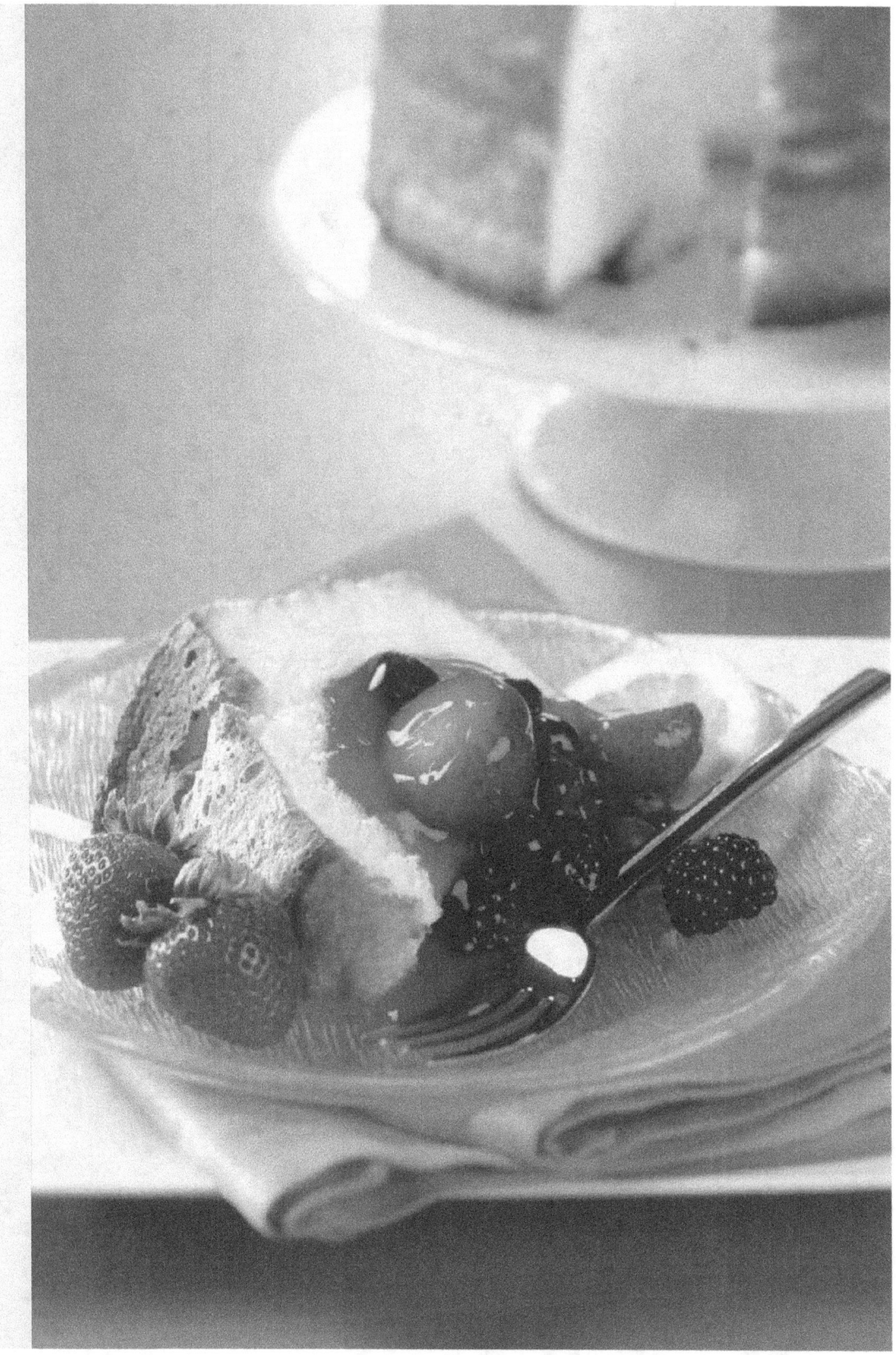

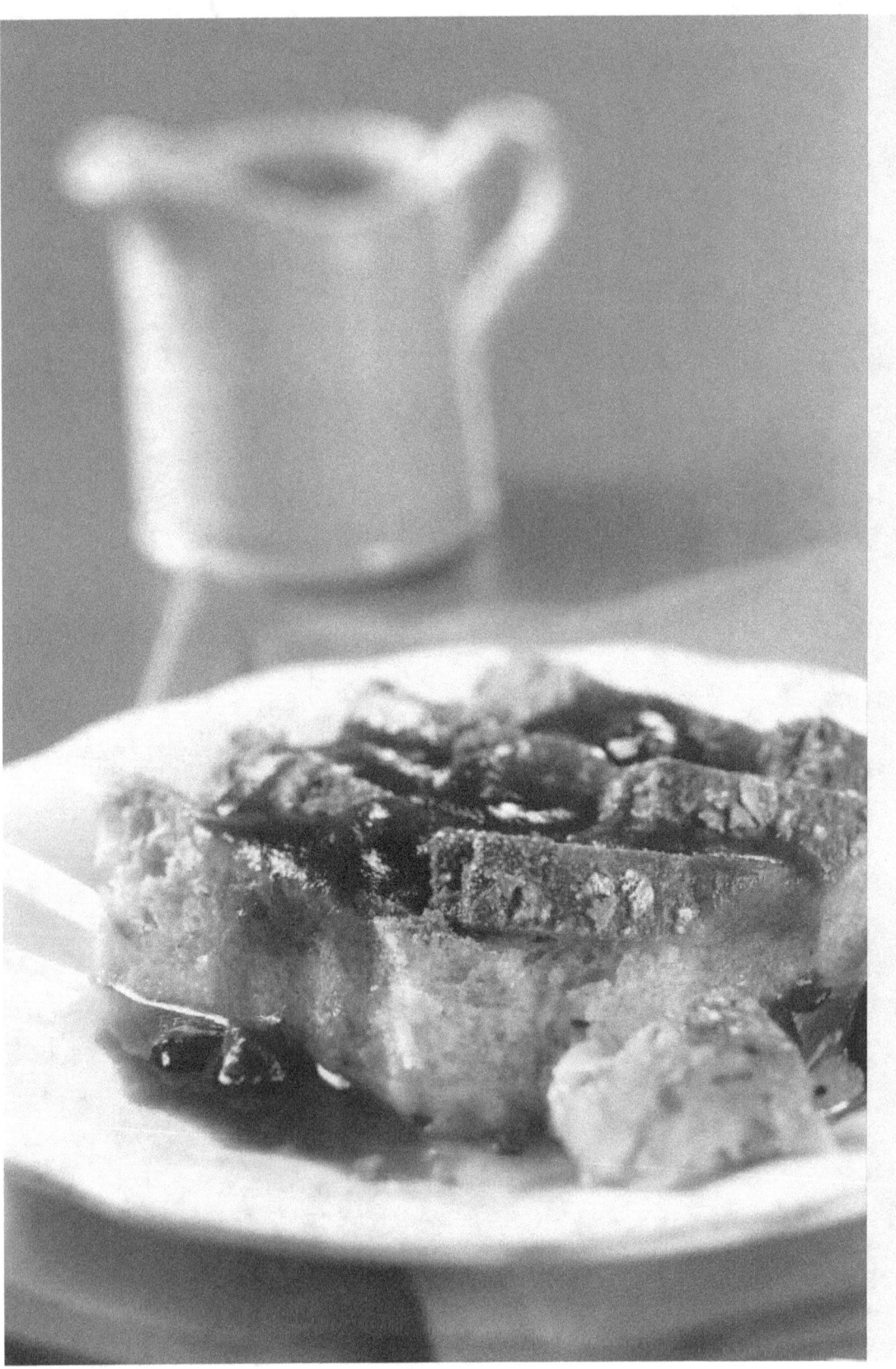

OLD-FASHIONED
BREAD PUDDING
with APPLE RAISIN SAUCE

1   Preheat the oven to 350° F. Spray an 8-inch x 8-inch baking dish with vegetable oil spray. Lay the slices of bread in the baking dish in two rows, overlapping them like shingles.

2   In a medium mixing bowl, beat together the egg, egg whites, milk, ¼ cup sugar, brown sugar, and vanilla. Pour the egg mixture over the bread.

3   In a small bowl, stir together the cinnamon, nutmeg, cloves, and 2 teaspoons sugar. Sprinkle the spiced sugar over the bread pudding. Bake the pudding for 30 to 35 minutes, until it has browned on top and is firm to the touch.

4   Serve warm or at room temperature, with warm apple-raisin sauce.

APPLE RAISIN SAUCE

Stir all the ingredients together in a medium saucepan. Bring to a simmer over low heat. Let the sauce simmer 5 minutes. Serve warm.

INGREDIENTS

10 slices whole wheat bread

1 egg

3 egg whites

1½ cups skim milk

¼ cup granulated sugar

¼ cup brown sugar

1 teaspoon vanilla extract

½ teaspoon cinnamon

¼ teaspoon nutmeg

¼ teaspoon cloves

2 teaspoons sugar

APPLE RAISIN SAUCE

1¼ cups apple juice

½ cup apple butter

2 tablespoons molasses

½ cup raisins

¼ teaspoon ground cinnamon

¼ teaspoon ground nutmeg

½ teaspoon orange peel (optional)

TO LEARN MORE ABOUT
NATIONAL CANCER INSTITUTE RESOURCES:

Contact the National Cancer Institute's
Cancer Information Service (CIS)

Toll free: 1-800-4-CANCER (1-800-433-6237)
TTY: 1-800-332-8615
Online: www.cancer.gov
Chat online: www.cancer.gov/help

NCI's CIS answers questions about cancer, clinical trials, and
cancer-related services and helps users find information on the
NCI Web site. Provides NCI printed materials.

www.ingramcontent.com/pod-product-compliance
Lightning Source LLC
Chambersburg PA
CBHW081621170526
45166CB00009B/3058